Low-fat
main meals

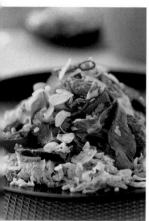 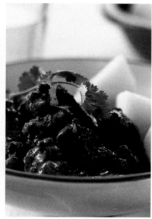 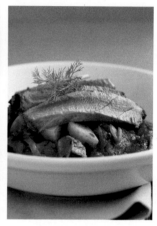

The Family Circle® Promise of Success

Welcome to the world of Confident Cooking, created for you in the
Family Circle® Test Kitchen, where recipes are double-tested by our team
of home economists to achieve a high standard of success.

MURDOCH
B O O K S

HEALTH AND WELLBEING

Low-fat eating can become a way of life and if combined with regular exercise will improve your health. Low-fat recipes with flavoursome ingredients are often more appealing than their high-fat counterparts.

HEALTHY EATING

It's never too late to change your eating habits and start repairing any damage you have done to your body. The body has an amazing capacity to heal itself, especially when fed a nutritious diet. A healthy diet doesn't mean eating bean sprouts and tofu for breakfast, lunch and dinner. Nor is it about being on an 'extreme diet' as these favour one nutrient over another, depriving the body of essential nutrients. The secret is to select from a wide range of foods in sensible proportions.

BALANCED DIET PYRAMID

The food pyramid opposite can be used as a guide to achieving a balanced diet. Eating a range of foods from each group will increase your chances of consuming a wide range of nutrients.

BENEFITS OF A HEALTHY DIET

- increases your energy

- helps maintain correct body weight

- reduces the risk of many common health problems

- improves ability to cope with stress

- helps maintain normal cholesterol and blood sugar levels

- keeps the immune system in shape

DAILY FAT INTAKE

Health authorities recommend we eat no more than 30% of our diet as fat, with less than 10% from saturated fat. For an average man, no more than 50–80 g of fat per day is recommended, and no more than 40–60 g for a woman.

COOKING TECHNIQUES

Some healthy cooking techniques are:

- use non-stick frying and saucepans as very little fat (if any) is needed

- lightly spray tins, frying pans and food with cooking oil spray, reducing the chance of adding too much oil

- steam vegetables to retain most of their nutrients and their colour

- cook stir-fry dishes quickly in small amounts of oil

- grill and barbecue to produce low-fat flavoursome meat

- bake some typically deep-fried dishes (fried chicken and nuggets) in the oven, using far less oil.

EXERCISE AND GOOD HEALTH

Exercise is important for good health. Excess fat in the diet is often stored as body fat. When exercise is combined with a lower fat intake, the body will use stored fat for energy.

THE BALANCED DIET PYRAMID

Eat least:
sugar, fats,
alcohol and salt

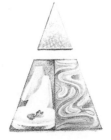

Eat moderately:
poultry, meat,
nuts, eggs and
dairy products

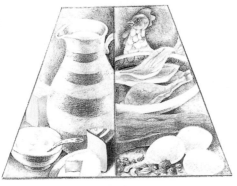

Eat most:
vegetables,
seafoods,
legumes,
cereals,
breads
and
fruits

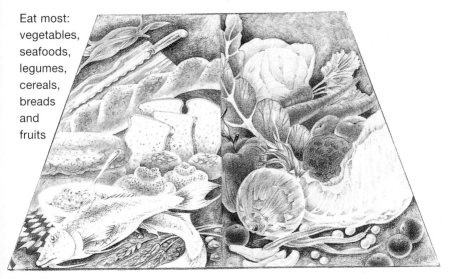

chicken and vegetable soup

PREP TIME: 25 MINUTES + OVERNIGHT
   REFRIGERATION
COOKING TIME: 3 HOURS
SERVES 6–8

Stock
2 tablespoons vegetable oil
1 large chicken (about 2 kg/4^1/2 lb),
   quartered
2 large onions, chopped
2 large carrots, chopped
1 celery stick, chopped
1 sprig of parsley
1 sprig of thyme
2 bay leaves

1 large leek, thinly sliced
1 large potato, cut into 2 cm
   (^{3}/4 inch) cubes
2 carrots, diced
150 g (5^1/2 oz) shelled peas
200 g (7 oz) green beans, trimmed and
   cut into 2 cm (^{3}/4 inch) lengths
100 g (3^1/2 oz) yellow beans, trimmed
   and cut into 2 cm (^{3}/4 inch) lengths
3 tablespoons chopped parsley
cayenne pepper, to garnish

1 Heat the oil in a large stockpot and brown the chicken pieces over medium heat for 10 minutes. Remove the chicken. Add the onion, carrot and celery to the pan and cook, stirring, for 6–8 minutes, or until golden brown. Return the chicken to the pan with the herbs, 3 litres (12 cups) water and ^{1}/2 teaspoon salt. Bring to a boil, reduce the heat and simmer, covered, for 2 hours, skimming the scum off the surface.

2 Remove the chicken pieces and cool the stock. Pour through a sieve into a large bowl. Discard the vegetables and herbs. Cover. Take the flesh off the chicken (discard the fat and bones) and shred into pieces. Cover. Refrigerate the stock and chicken overnight. Remove the layer of fat from the top of the stock.

3 Bring the stock to the boil in a saucepan. Add the leek, potato and carrot and simmer for 30 minutes, or until tender. Add the chicken, peas and beans and simmer for 15 minutes, or until the vegetables are tender. Stir in the parsley. Season with salt and cayenne pepper.

NUTRITION PER SERVE (8): Fat 6 g; Carbohydrate 8 g; Protein 20.5 g; Dietary Fibre 3 g; Cholesterol 57 mg; 700 kJ (165 Cal)

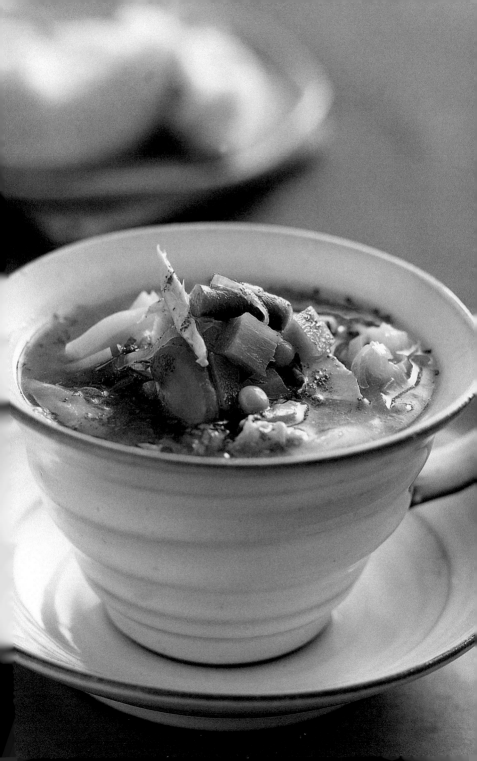

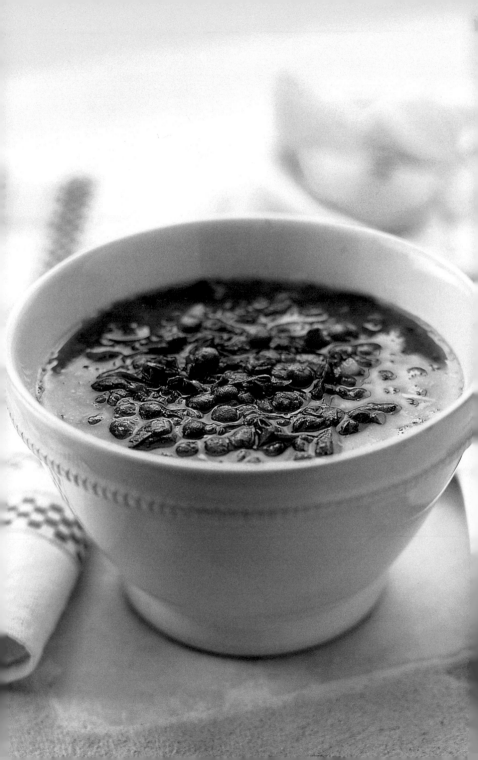

lentil and silverbeet soup

PREP TIME: 15 MINUTES
COOKING TIME: 1 HOUR 10 MINUTES
SERVES 6

280 g (1 1/2 cups) brown lentils, washed
1 litre (4 cups) chicken stock
850 g (1 lb 14 oz) silverbeet
3 tablespoons olive oil
1 large onion, finely chopped
4 garlic cloves, crushed
25 g (1/2 cup) finely chopped coriander
4 tablespoons lemon juice
lemon wedges, to serve

NUTRITION PER SERVE: Fat 15 g; Carbohydrate 20 g; Protein 38 g; Dietary Fibre 11 g; Cholesterol 83 mg; 1782 kJ (425 Cal)

1 Put the lentils in a large saucepan with the stock and 1 litre (4 cups) water. Bring to the boil, then reduce the heat and simmer, covered, for 1 hour.

2 Remove the stems from the silverbeet and shred the leaves. Heat the oil in a saucepan over medium heat and cook the onion for 2–3 minutes, or until transparent. Add the garlic and cook for 1 minute. Add the silverbeet and toss for 2–3 minutes, or until wilted. Stir the mixture into the lentils.

3 Add the chopped coriander and the lemon juice, then season and cover. Simmer for 15–20 minutes. Serve with the lemon wedges.

ravioli broth with lemon and baby spinach

PREP TIME: 15 MINUTES + OVERNIGHT
    REFRIGERATION
COOKING TIME: 3 HOURS 35 MINUTES
SERVES 4

1.5 litres (6 cups) chicken stock
350 g (12 oz) fresh veal ravioli
2 strips lemon zest (6 cm/2 1/2 inches long), white pith removed
150 g (5 1/2 oz) baby English spinach leaves, stems removed
1/2 teaspoon lemon oil
1–2 tablespoons lemon juice
40 g (1/2 cup) shaved Parmesan, to serve (optional)

NUTRITION PER SERVE: Fat 11.5 g; Carbohydrate 36 g; Protein 20 g; Dietary Fibre 4 g; Cholesterol 32.5 mg; 1360 kJ (325 Cal)

1 Pour the stock into a large saucepan and bring to the boil. Add the veal ravioli and lemon zest and cook for 3–5 minutes, or until the ravioli floats to the top and is tender.

2 Discard the zest. Stir in the spinach leaves and season. Just before serving, stir in the lemon oil, to taste, and lemon juice. Serve with Parmesan, if desired.

chicken and spinach risoni soup

PREP TIME: 15 MINUTES
COOKING TIME: 35 MINUTES
SERVES 4

1 tablespoon olive oil
1 leek, quartered lengthways and
   thinly sliced
2 garlic cloves, crushed
1 teaspoon ground cumin
1.5 litres (6 cups) chicken stock
2 chicken breast fillets
   (about 200 g/7 oz each)
200 g (1 cup) risoni (see Note)
150 g (5¹/2 oz) baby English spinach
   leaves, roughly chopped
1 tablespoon chopped dill
2 teaspoons lemon juice

NUTRITION PER SERVE: Fat 13.5 g; Carbohydrate 39 g;
Protein 38 g; Dietary Fibre 3.5 g; Cholesterol 82.5 mg;
1815 kJ (435 Cal)

1 Heat the oil in a large saucepan over a low heat. Add the leek and cook for 8–10 minutes, or until soft. Add the garlic and cumin and cook for 1 minute. Pour the chicken stock into the pan, increase the heat to high and bring to the boil. Reduce the heat to low, add the chicken fillets and simmer, covered, for 8 minutes. Remove the chicken from the broth with a slotted spoon, allow it to cool slightly, then shred it into small pieces.

2 Stir the risoni into the broth and simmer for 12 minutes, or until *al dente*.

3 Return the chicken to the broth and add the chopped spinach and dill. Simmer for 2 minutes, or until the spinach has wilted.

4 Just before serving, stir in the lemon juice and season to taste with salt and freshly ground black pepper.

note: Risoni is a rice-shaped pasta that is usually used in soups.

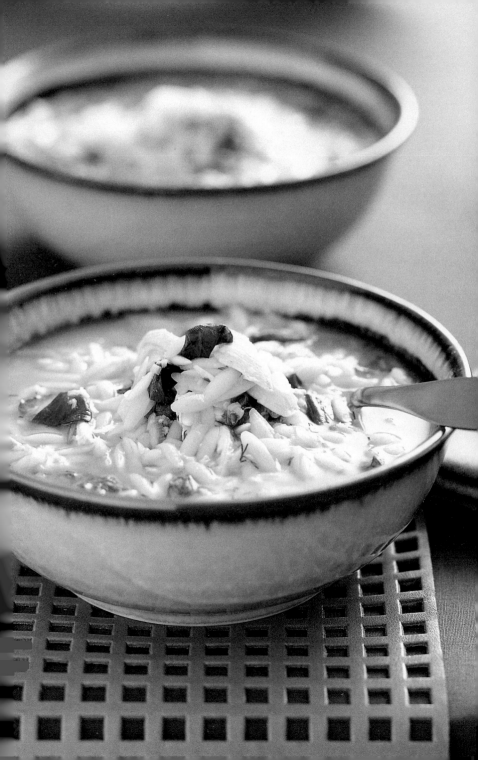

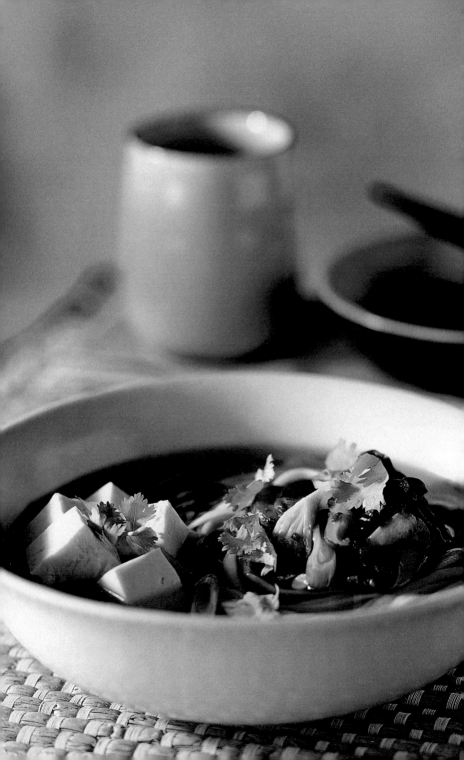

tofu and asian mushroom noodle soup

PREP TIME: 20 MINUTES
COOKING TIME: 15 MINUTES
SERVES 4

2 dried Chinese mushrooms
10 g (1/4 oz) dried black fungus
1 tablespoon vegetable oil
6 spring onions (scallions), thickly sliced
    on the diagonal
1 red chilli, seeded and chopped
60 g (2 1/4 oz) oyster mushrooms, sliced
60 g (2 1/4 oz) Swiss brown mushrooms,
    sliced
1 1/2 tablespoons dashi granules
3 tablespoons light soy sauce
1 1/2 tablespoons mirin
125 g (4 1/2 oz) dried wheat noodles
200 g (7 oz) water spinach or spinach, cut
    into 4 cm (1 1/2 inch) slices
300 g (10 1/2 oz) firm tofu, cut into
    2 cm (3/4 inch) cubes
10 g (1/3 cup) coriander (cilantro) leaves

NUTRITION PER SERVE: Fat 10.5 g; Carbohydrate 26 g;
Protein 17 g; Dietary Fibre 5.5 g; Cholesterol 0 mg;
1105 kJ (265 Cal)

1 Soak the Chinese mushrooms in 250 ml (1 cup) hot water to soften. Squeeze dry and reserve the liquid. Discard the stalks and finely chop the caps. Cover the black fungus in hot water and soak until soft. Drain.

2 Heat the oil in a large saucepan or wok. Cook the Chinese mushrooms, black fungus, spring onion and chilli over high heat for 1 minute. Add the oyster and Swiss brown mushrooms and cook for 2 minutes.

3 Stir in the dashi granules, soy sauce, mirin, reserved mushroom liquid and 1.5 litres (6 cups) water. Bring to the boil, then stir in the noodles. Cook over medium heat for 5 minutes, or until soft.

4 Add the water spinach and cook for 2 minutes, then add the tofu and coriander. Serve at once.

note: Dashi granules can be bought at Japanese shops and at some supermarkets. Water spinach can be bought at Asian grocery shops.

prawn gumbo

PREP TIME: 15 MINUTES
COOKING TIME: 1 HOUR
SERVES 4

2 tablespoons olive oil
1 large onion, finely chopped
3 garlic cloves, crushed
1 red capsicum (pepper), chopped
4 bacon rashers, chopped
1 1/2 teaspoons dried thyme
2 teaspoons dried oregano
1 teaspoon paprika
1/2 teaspoon cayenne pepper
3 tablespoons sherry
1 litre (4 cups) fish stock
100 g (1/2 cup) long-grain rice
2 bay leaves
400 g (14 oz) can chopped tomatoes
150 g (5 1/2 oz) okra, thinly sliced
   (see Note)
850 g (1 lb 14 oz) raw medium prawns
   (shrimp), peeled and deveined
3 tablespoons finely chopped parsley

NUTRITION PER SERVE: Fat 15 g; Carbohydrate 31 g;
Protein 61 g; Dietary Fibre 5 g; Cholesterol 341.5 mg;
2175 kJ (520 Cal)

1 Heat the oil in a large saucepan over low heat. Cook the onion, garlic, capsicum and bacon for 5 minutes, or until soft. Stir in the herbs and spices. Season. Add the sherry and cook until evaporated, then add the stock and 500 ml (2 cups) water. Bring to a boil. Add the rice and bay leaves, reduce the heat and simmer, covered, for 20 minutes.

2 Add the tomato and okra. Simmer, covered, for 20–25 minutes. Stir in the prawns and parsley and simmer for 5 minutes, or until the prawns are cooked through.

note: Okra is a slender, five-sided pod that contains numerous white seeds. When cooked, okra releases a sticky, gelatinous substance that serves to thicken soups and stews. Buy pods that are tender and healthy green in colour. If too ripe, the pod will feel very sticky.

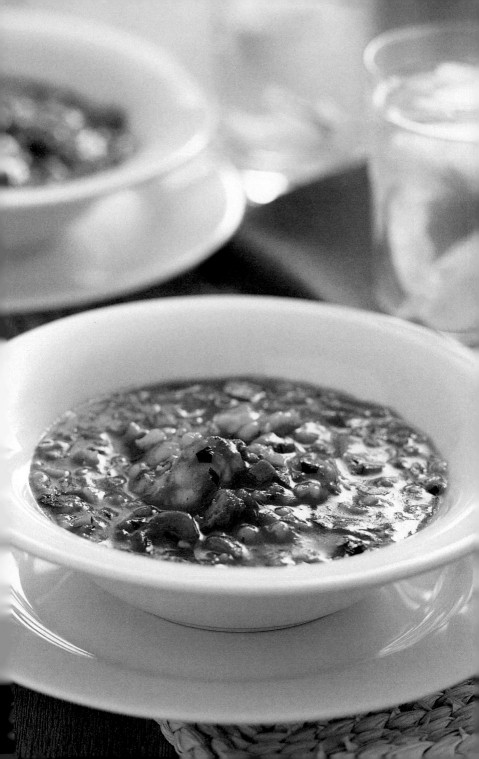

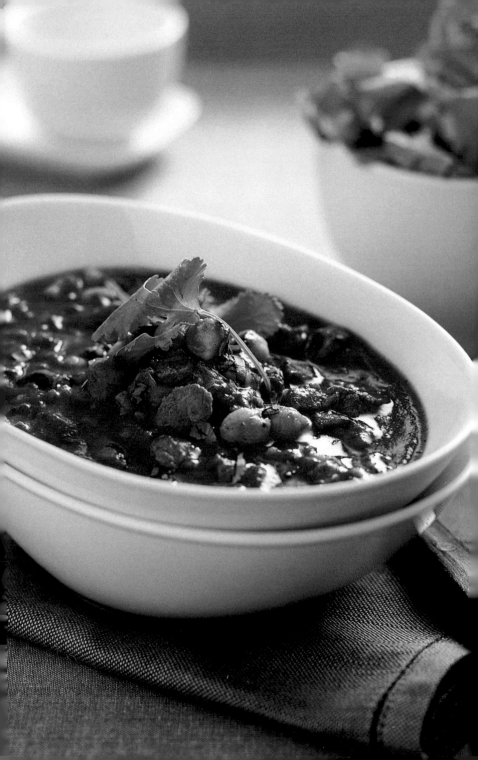

moroccan lamb, chickpea and coriander soup

PREP TIME: 15 MINUTES + OVERNIGHT
   SOAKING
COOKING TIME: 2 HOURS 15 MINUTES
SERVES 4–6

165 g ($^3/_4$ cup) dried chickpeas
1 tablespoon olive oil
850 g (1 lb 14 oz) boned lamb leg,
   cut into 1 cm ($^1/_2$ inch) cubes
1 onion, chopped
2 garlic cloves, crushed
$^1/_2$ teaspoon ground cinnamon
$^1/_2$ teaspoon ground turmeric
$^1/_2$ teaspoon ground ginger
4 tablespoons chopped coriander (cilantro)
2 x 400 g (14 oz) cans chopped tomatoes
1 litre (4 cups) chicken stock
160 g ($^2/_3$ cup) dried red lentils, rinsed
coriander (cilantro) leaves, to garnish

NUTRITION PER SERVE (6): Fat 9.5 g; Carbohydrate 22 g;
Protein 29 g; Dietary Fibre 7.5 g; Cholesterol 51 mg;
1200 kJ (285 Cal)

1 Soak the chickpeas in cold water overnight. Drain, and rinse well.

2 Heat the oil in a large saucepan over high heat and brown the lamb in batches for 2–3 minutes. Reduce the heat to medium, return the lamb to the pan with the onion and garlic and cook for 5 minutes. Add the spices, season and cook for 2 minutes. Add the coriander, tomato, stock and 500 ml (2 cups) water and bring to the boil over high heat.

3 Add the lentils and chickpeas and simmer, covered, over low heat for 1 hour 30 minutes. Uncover and cook for 30 minutes, or until the lamb is tender and the soup is thick. Season. Garnish with coriander.

hot and sour lime soup with beef

PREP TIME: 20 MINUTES
COOKING TIME: 30 MINUTES
SERVES 4

1 litre (4 cups) beef stock
2 stems lemon grass, white part only, halved
3 garlic cloves, halved
2.5 x 2.5 cm (1 inch x 1 inch) piece fresh ginger, sliced
100 g ($3^1/2$ oz) coriander (cilantro), leaves and stalks separated
4 spring onions (scallions), thinly sliced on the diagonal
2 strips lime zest
2 star anise
3 small red chillies, seeded and finely chopped
500 g (1 lb 2 oz) fillet steak, trimmed
2 tablespoons fish sauce
1 tablespoon grated palm sugar or soft brown sugar
2 tablespoons lime juice
coriander (cilantro) leaves, extra, to garnish

NUTRITION PER SERVE: Fat 7 g; Carbohydrate 7 g; Protein 31 g; Dietary Fibre 0.5 g; Cholesterol 84 mg; 900 kJ (215 Cal)

1 Put the beef stock, lemon grass, garlic, ginger, coriander stalks, 2 spring onions, lime zest, star anise, 1 teaspoon chopped chilli and 1 litre (4 cups) water in a saucepan. Bring to a boil and simmer, covered, for 25 minutes. Strain and return the liquid to the pan.

2 Heat a ridged chargrill pan (griddle) until very hot. Brush lightly with olive oil and sear the steak on both sides until browned on the outside, but very rare in the centre.

3 Reheat the soup, adding the fish sauce and palm sugar. Season with salt and black pepper. Add the lime juice to taste (you may want more than 2 tablespoons)—you should achieve a hot and sour flavour.

4 Add the remaining spring onion and the chopped coriander leaves to the soup. Slice the beef across the grain into thin strips. Curl the strips into a decorative pattern, then place in the centre of four deep wide serving bowls. Pour the soup over the beef and garnish with the remaining chilli and a few extra coriander leaves.

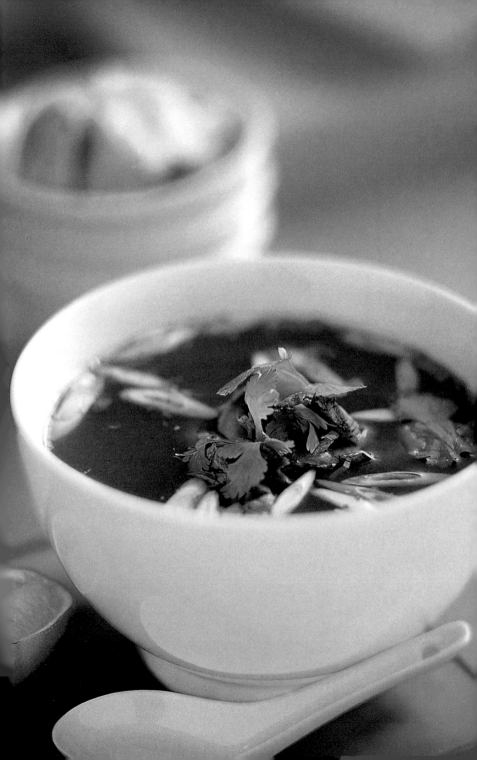

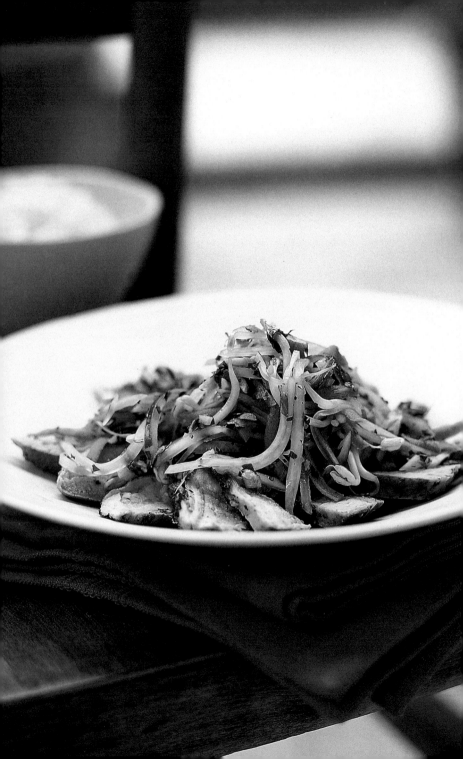

thai pork tenderloin and green mango salad

PREP TIME: 45 MINUTES + 2 HOURS
    REFRIGERATION
COOKING TIME: 10 MINUTES
SERVES 4 AS A MAIN (6 AS AN ENTRÉE)

2 stems lemon grass (white part only),
    thinly sliced
1 garlic clove
2 red Asian shallots
1 tablespoon coarsely chopped fresh ginger
1 red bird's-eye chilli, seeded
1 tablespoon fish sauce
15 g ($^1/_2$ cup) coriander (cilantro) leaves
1 teaspoon grated lime zest
1 tablespoon lime juice
2 tablespoons oil
2 pork tenderloins, trimmed

Dressing

1 large red chilli, seeded and finely chopped
2 garlic cloves, finely chopped
3 coriander (cilantro) roots, finely chopped
1 tablespoon grated palm sugar or soft
    brown sugar
2 tablespoons fish sauce
3 tablespoons lime juice

Salad

2 green mangoes or 1 small green papaya,
    peeled and cut into julienne strips
1 carrot, grated
45 g ($^1/_2$ cup) bean sprouts
$^1/_2$ red onion, thinly sliced
3 tablespoons chopped mint
3 tablespoons chopped coriander (cilantro)
3 tablespoons chopped Vietnamese mint

1 Place the lemon grass, garlic, shallots, ginger, chilli, fish sauce, coriander, lime zest, lime juice and oil in a blender or food processor and process until a coarse paste forms. Transfer to a non-metallic dish. Coat the pork in the marinade, cover and refrigerate for at least 2 hours, but no longer than 4 hours.

2 To make the salad dressing, mix all the ingredients together in a bowl.

3 To make the salad, combine all the salad ingredients in a large bowl.

4 Preheat a grill or chargrill pan (griddle) and cook the pork over medium heat for 4–5 minutes each side, or until cooked through. Remove from the heat and rest for 5 minutes before slicing.

5 Toss the dressing and salad together. Season to taste with salt and cracked black pepper. Arrange the sliced pork in a circle in the centre of each plate and top with salad. To make this a main course, serve with steamed jasmine rice, if desired.

NUTRITION PER SERVE (4): Fat 14 g; Carbohydrate 20 g; Protein 60 g; Dietary Fibre 3 g; Cholesterol 122 mg; 1860 kJ (444 Cal)

thai beef salad

PREP TIME: 30 MINUTES + 15 MINUTES
  REFRIGERATION
COOKING TIME: 10 MINUTES
SERVES 4

1 tablespoon oil
2 x 250 g (9 oz) pieces rump steak
3^{1}/$_{2}$ tablespoons lime juice
2 tablespoons fish sauce
1 teaspoon grated palm sugar or soft
  brown sugar
2 garlic cloves, crushed
1 stem lemon grass, white part only,
  thinly sliced
2 small red chillies, thinly sliced
4 red Asian shallots, thinly sliced
15–20 mint leaves
15 g (^{1}/$_{2}$ cup) coriander (cilantro) leaves
125 g (4^{1}/$_{2}$ oz) cherry tomatoes, halved
1 Lebanese (short) cucumber, halved
  lengthways and thinly sliced
180 g (3 cups) shredded Chinese cabbage
20 g (^{1}/$_{4}$ cup) bought Asian fried onions
  (see Note)
1 tablespoon bought Asian fried garlic (see
  Note)
40 g (^{1}/$_{4}$ cup) crushed peanuts, to garnish
  (optional)

NUTRITION PER SERVE: Fat 11 g; Carbohydrate 5 g;
Protein 32 g; Dietary Fibre 3.5 g; Cholesterol 80 mg;
1040 kJ (250 Cal)

1 Heat the oil in a large, non-stick frying pan over high heat. Cook the steak for 4 minutes each side, then remove and cool.

2 Combine the lime juice, fish sauce, palm sugar, garlic, lemon grass and chilli and stir to dissolve the sugar. Add the shallots, mint and coriander. Thinly slice the beef across the grain, and toss through the mixture. Chill for 15 minutes. Add the tomato and cucumber and toss. Arrange the cabbage on a serving platter and top with the beef mixture. Sprinkle with the fried onion, garlic and peanuts, if desired.

note: Asian fried onions and Asian fried garlic can be bought from Asian stores and some supermarkets.

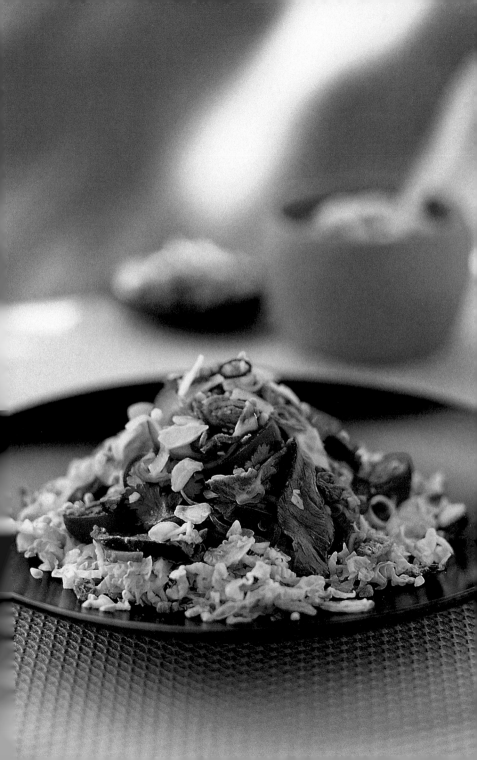

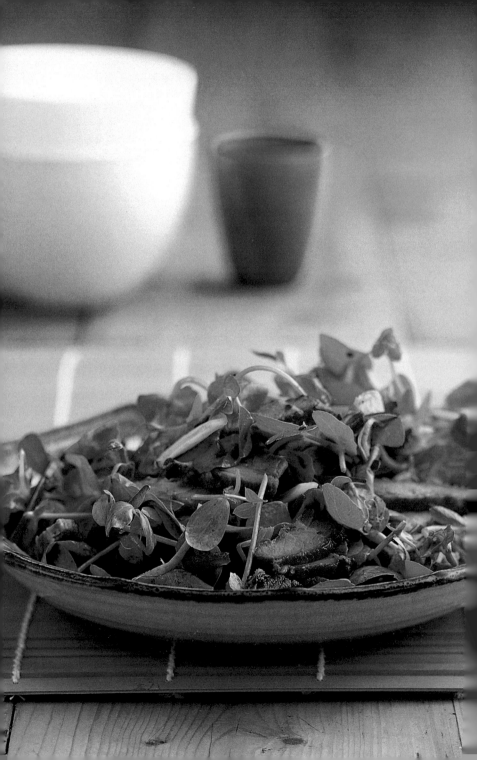

asian pork salad

PREP TIME: 15 MINUTES
COOKING TIME: 2 MINUTES
SERVES 4

2 teaspoons rice vinegar
1 small red chilli, finely chopped
2 tablespoons light soy sauce
1 teaspoon julienned fresh ginger
$1/4$ teaspoon sesame oil
1 star anise
2 teaspoons lime juice
250 g (9 oz) Asian roasted pork (see Note)
100 g ($3^1/2$ oz) snow pea (mangetout)
   shoots
2 spring onions (scallions), thinly sliced
   on the diagonal
$1/2$ red capsicum (pepper), thinly sliced

NUTRITION PER SERVE: Fat 10 g; Carbohydrate 10 g;
Protein 17 g; Dietary Fibre 3.5 g; Cholesterol 39.5 mg;
810 kJ (195 Cal)

1 For the dressing, combine the vinegar, chilli, soy sauce, ginger, sesame oil, star anise and lime juice in a small saucepan. Gently warm for 2 minutes, or until just about to come to the boil, then set aside to cool. Once it is cool, remove the star anise.

2 Thinly slice the pork and place in a serving bowl. Pick over the shoots, discarding any brown or broken ones, and add to the pork. Add the spring onion and capsicum, pour on the dressing, and toss well.

note: Pieces of Asian roast pork can be bought at Asian restaurants that sell roast meats.

tandoori lamb salad

PREP TIME: 20 MINUTES + OVERNIGHT
   MARINATING
COOKING TIME: 15 MINUTES
SERVES 4

250 g (1 cup) low-fat plain yoghurt
2 garlic cloves, crushed
2 teaspoons grated fresh ginger
2 teaspoons ground turmeric
2 teaspoons garam masala
$1/4$ teaspoon paprika
2 teaspoons ground coriander
red food colouring (optional)
500 g (1 lb 2 oz) lean lamb fillets
4 tablespoons lemon juice
$1^1/2$ teaspoons chopped coriander
   (cilantro)
1 teaspoon chopped mint
150 g ($5^1/2$ oz) mixed salad leaves
1 large mango, cut into strips
2 cucumbers, cut into matchsticks

NUTRITION PER SERVE: Fat 6.5 g; Carbohydrate 8 g;
Protein 30 g; Dietary Fibre 2 g; Cholesterol 90 mg;
965 kJ (230 Cal)

1 Mix the yoghurt, garlic, ginger and spices in a bowl, add a little colouring, if desired, and toss with the lamb to coat. Cover and refrigerate overnight.

2 Grill the lamb on a foil-lined baking tray under a high heat for 7 minutes each side, or until the marinade starts to brown. Set aside for 5 minutes before serving.

3 Mix the lemon juice, chopped coriander and mint, then season. Toss with the salad leaves, mango and cucumber, then arrange on plates. Slice the lamb and serve over the salad.

pictured: asian pork salad

prawn and saffron potato salad

PREP TIME: 15 MINUTES
COOKING TIME: 30 MINUTES
SERVES 4

4 tablespoons olive oil
450 g (1 lb) new potatoes, cut in half
1/4 teaspoon saffron threads, crushed
16 raw medium prawns (shrimp), peeled
   and deveined, with the tails intact
1 garlic clove, crushed
1 bird's eye chilli, seeded and finely
   chopped
1 teaspoon grated lime zest
3 tablespoons lime juice
200 g (7 oz) baby rocket (arugula)

NUTRITION PER SERVE: Fat 12.5 g; Carbohydrate 17 g;
Protein 19 g; Dietary Fibre 3.5 g; Cholesterol 106 mg;
1065 kJ (255 Cal)

1 Preheat the oven to 180°C (350°F/ Gas 4). Heat 2 tablespoons of the oil in a frying pan and brown the potatoes. Transfer to a roasting tin and toss gently with the saffron and some salt and pepper. Bake for 25 minutes, or until tender.

2 Heat a chargrill pan (griddle) over medium heat. Toss the prawns with the garlic, chilli, lime zest and 1 tablespoon of the oil in a small bowl. Grill the prawns for 2 minutes each side, or until pink and cooked.

3 In a small jar, shake the lime juice and the remaining oil together. Season.

4 Put the potatoes on a plate, top with the rocket and prawns and drizzle with the dressing.

tuna and bean salad

PREP TIME: 20 MINUTES + 10 MINUTES
   REFRIGERATION
COOKING TIME: 5 MINUTES
SERVES 4

100 g (3 1/2 oz) green beans, chopped
400 g (14 oz) can butter (lima) beans,
   rinsed and drained
425 g (15 oz) can tuna in brine, drained
200 g (7 oz) cherry tomatoes, quartered
1 red onion, thinly sliced
100 g (3 1/2 oz) mixed salad leaves
100 g (3 1/2 oz) baby rocket (arugula)
   leaves

Dressing

1 tablespoon extra virgin olive oil
3 tablespoons lemon juice
1 teaspoon honey
2 garlic cloves, crushed
2 tablespoons chopped dill

NUTRITION PER SERVE: Fat 7 g; Carbohydrate 7.5 g;
Protein 24.5 g; Dietary Fibre 4.5 g; Cholesterol 43 mg;
815 kJ (195 Cal)

1 Steam the green beans until tender, rinse under cold water and drain. Place the green and butter beans, tuna, tomato and onion in a bowl, and toss well.

2 To make the dressing, whisk all the ingredients together. Pour the dressing over the tuna mixture, cover and refrigerate for 10 minutes.

3 Combine the salad leaves and rocket, and arrange on a salad platter. Top with the tuna mixture and serve.

pictured: prawn and saffron potato salad

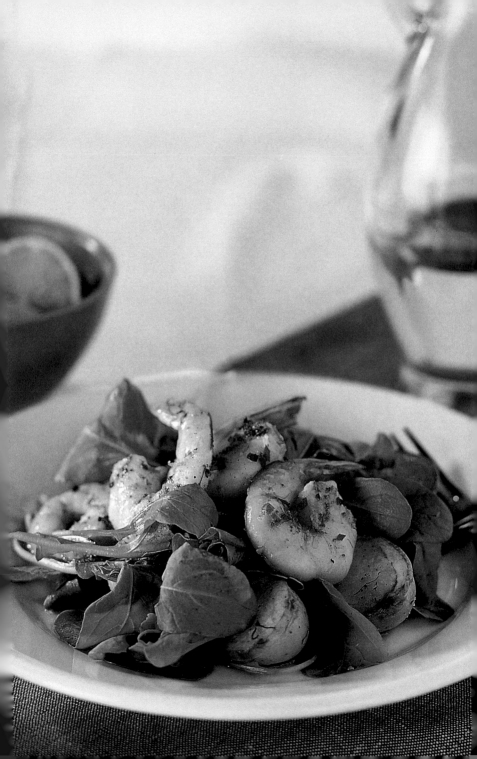

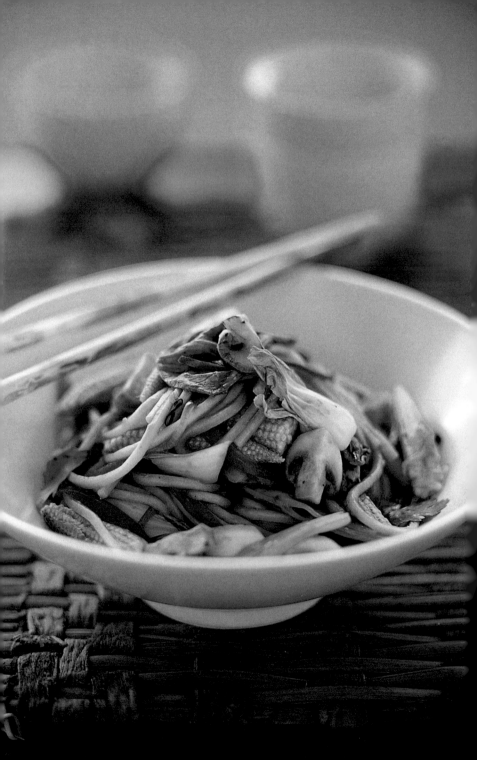

vegetable and noodle stir-fry

PREP TIME: 25 MINUTES
COOKING TIME: 10 MINUTES
SERVES 4

350 g ($^3/_4$ lb) fresh hokkien (egg) noodles
1 teaspoon sesame oil
2 tablespoons vegetable oil
1 red onion, halved and thinly sliced
3 garlic cloves, crushed
3 x 3 cm ($1^1/_4$ x $1^1/_4$ inch) piece fresh
    ginger, julienned
5 spring onions (scallions), cut into
    5 cm (2 inch) lengths
1 small red chilli, seeded and
    finely chopped
3 star anise
1 small red capsicum (pepper), thinly sliced
100 g ($3^1/_2$ oz) snow peas (mangetout),
    trimmed and halved diagonally
100 g ($3^1/_2$ oz) open cap mushrooms,
    quartered
500 g (1 lb 2 oz) baby bok choy (pak choi),
    trimmed, leaves separated, cut into
    5 cm (2 inch) lengths
115 g ($^1/_4$ lb) baby corn, halved diagonally
2 teaspoons cornflour (cornstarch)
100 ml ($3^1/_2$ fl oz) Chinese barbecue sauce
    (char sui)
2 tablespoons Chinese rice wine
    (see Note)
15 g ($^1/_2$ cup) coriander (cilantro) leaves

NUTRITION PER SERVE: Fat 12.5 g; Carbohydrate 69 g; Protein 14 g; Dietary Fibre 7.5 g; Cholesterol 11.5 mg; 1880 kJ (450 Cal)

1 Put the noodles in a large heatproof bowl, cover with boiling water and soak for 5 minutes. Use a fork to gently separate the noodles, then drain well. Toss with the sesame oil.

2 Heat a wok over high heat. Add the vegetable oil and swirl to coat. Add the red onion, garlic, ginger, spring onion and chilli and stir-fry for 1 minute. Add the star anise, capsicum, snow peas, mushrooms, bok choy and baby corn and stir-fry for 2–3 minutes.

3 Mix the cornflour with 1 teaspoon cold water. Add to the wok with the barbecue sauce and Chinese rice wine. Bring to the boil and cook for 1 minute, or until the ingredients are coated and the sauce thickens slightly. Stir in the coriander leaves and serve immediately.

note: Chinese rice wine can be bought from Asian food stores and some large supermarkets. Otherwise you can use dry sherry.

tuna steaks on coriander noodles

PREP TIME: 15 MINUTES
COOKING TIME: 10 MINUTES
SERVES 4

3 tablespoons lime juice
2 tablespoons fish sauce
2 tablespoons sweet chilli sauce
2 teaspoons grated palm sugar or soft
  brown sugar
1 teaspoon sesame oil
1 garlic clove, finely chopped
1 tablespoon virgin olive oil
4 tuna steaks (150 g/5^1/$_2$ oz each), at
  room temperature
200 g (7 oz) dried thin wheat noodles
6 spring onions (scallions), thinly sliced
25 g (^{1}/$_2$ cup) chopped coriander (cilantro)
lime wedges, to garnish

NUTRITION PER SERVE: Fat 10 g; Carbohydrate 5 g; Protein 32 g; Dietary Fibre 1 g; Cholesterol 105 mg; 1030 kJ (245 Cal)

1 To make the dressing, place the lime juice, fish sauce, chilli sauce, sugar, sesame oil and garlic in a small bowl and mix together.

2 Heat the olive oil in a chargrill pan (griddle). Add the tuna steaks and cook over high heat for 2 minutes each side, or until cooked to your liking. Transfer the tuna to a warm plate, cover and keep warm.

3 Place the noodles in a large saucepan of lightly salted, rapidly boiling water and return to the boil. Cook for 4 minutes, or until the noodles are tender. Drain well. Add half the dressing and half the spring onion and coriander to the noodles and gently toss together.

4 Either cut the tuna into even cubes or slice it.

5 Place the noodles on serving plates and top with the tuna. Mix the remaining dressing with the spring onion and coriander and drizzle over the tuna. Garnish with lime wedges.

note: If you prefer, you can serve the tuna steaks whole rather than cutting them into cubes. If serving whole, they would look better served with the noodles on the side.

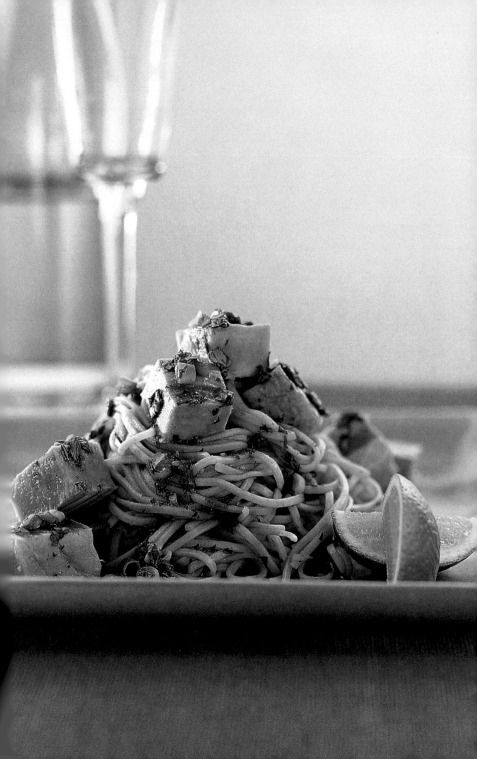

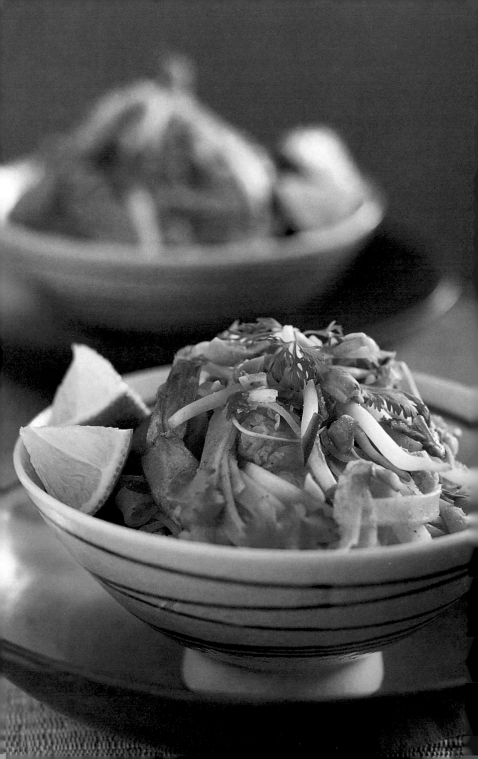

thai-style noodles

PREP TIME: 40 MINUTES
COOKING TIME: 10 MINUTES
SERVES 4–6

250 g (9 oz) flat dried rice stick noodles
1 small red chilli, chopped
2 garlic cloves, chopped
2 spring onions (scallions), sliced
1 tablespoon tamarind purée, combined
    with 1 tablespoon water (see Note)
1$\frac{1}{2}$ tablespoons grated palm sugar or soft
    brown sugar
2 tablespoons fish sauce
2 tablespoons lime juice
2 tablespoons oil
2 eggs, beaten
150 g (5$\frac{1}{2}$ oz) pork fillet, thinly sliced
8 raw large prawns (shrimp), peeled,
    deveined and tails intact
100 g (3$\frac{1}{2}$ oz) fried tofu, julienned
90 g (1 cup) bean sprouts
40 g ($\frac{1}{4}$ cup) chopped roasted peanuts
3 tablespoons coriander (cilantro) leaves
1 lime, cut into wedges or cheeks

NUTRITION PER SERVE (6): Fat 8.5 g; Carbohydrate 15 g;
Protein 14 g; Dietary Fibre 0.5 g; Cholesterol 110 mg;
812 kJ (194 Cal)

1 Soak the noodles in warm water for 10 minutes. Drain.

2 Pound the chilli, garlic and spring onion in a mortar and pestle. Gradually blend in the tamarind mixture, sugar, fish sauce and lime juice.

3 Heat a wok until very hot, add 1 tablespoon of the oil and swirl to coat. Add the egg, swirl to coat and cook for 1–2 minutes, or until set and cooked. Remove and shred.

4 Heat the remaining oil, stir in the chilli mixture and stir-fry for 30 seconds. Add the pork and stir-fry for 2 minutes, or until tender. Add the prawns and stir-fry for another 1 minute.

5 Stir in the drained noodles, egg, tofu and half the bean sprouts and toss to heat through.

6 Serve immediately topped with the peanuts, coriander, lime and remaining bean sprouts.

note: Tamarind has a sweet–sour flavour. The purée is available in jars in Asian food stores or the Asian section of some supermarkets.

pasta with grilled capsicum

PREP TIME: 15 MINUTES
COOKING TIME: 15 MINUTES
SERVES 4–6

400 g (14 oz) pasta gnocchi
6 large red capsicums (peppers), halved
2 tablespoons olive oil
1 onion, thinly sliced
3 garlic cloves, finely chopped
2 tablespoons shredded basil
whole basil leaves, to garnish
shaved Parmesan cheese, to serve (optional)

NUTRITION PER SERVE (6): Fat 7 g; Carbohydrate 62 g; Protein 11 g; Dietary Fibre 4 g; Cholesterol 0 mg; 1515 kJ (360 Cal)

1 Cook the pasta in a large pan of rapidly boiling salted water until *al dente.*

2 Cut the capsicums into large flattish pieces. Cook, skin-side-up, under a hot grill until the skin blackens and blisters. Put in a plastic bag and cool, then peel.

3 Heat the oil in a large frying pan, add the onion and garlic and cook over medium heat for 5 minutes, or until soft. Cut one capsicum into thin strips and add it to the onion mixture.

4 Chop the remaining capsicum, then purée in the food processor until smooth. Add to the onion mixture and cook over low heat for 5 minutes, or until warmed through.

5 Toss the sauce through the pasta. Season, then stir in the shredded basil. Garnish with basil leaves and serve with Parmesan if desired.

pasta with slow-roast tomato sauce

PREP TIME: 15 MINUTES
COOKING TIME: 3 HOURS 10 MINUTES
SERVES 4–6

500 g (1 lb 2 oz) penne rigate
2 kg (4 lb 8 oz) ripe Roma (plum) tomatoes
1 large red onion, chopped
4 garlic cloves, finely chopped
1 tablespoon finely chopped thyme
2 teaspoons soft brown sugar
1 tablespoon good-quality balsamic vinegar
4 tablespoons olive oil
shaved Parmesan cheese, to serve

NUTRITION PER SERVE (6): Fat 12 g; Carbohydrate 8.5 g; Protein 3.5 g; Dietary Fibre 4.5 g; Cholesterol 0 mg; 665 kJ (160 Cal)

1 Cook the pasta in a large pan of rapidly boiling salted water until *al dente.*

2 Preheat the oven to 180°C (350°F/ Gas 4). Cut the tomatoes into large chunks and put them in a large roasting tin. Add the onion, garlic, thyme, sugar, vinegar, olive oil and a generous amount of salt and freshly ground black pepper, then toss together until well combined.

3 Roast the tomatoes, stirring every 20 minutes or so, for 2¹/₂–3 hours, or until the tomatoes are slightly caramelized and breaking down to form a chunky sauce. Season to taste, then toss with the hot pasta. Sprinkle with some Parmesan before serving.

pictured: pasta with grilled capsicum

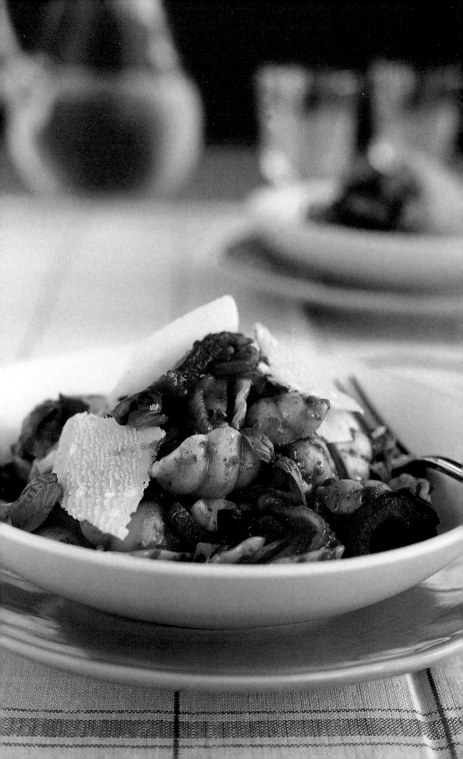

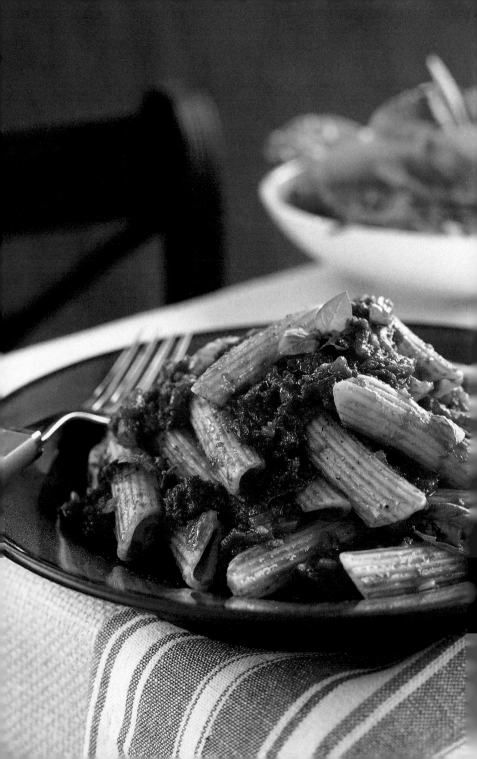

pasta pomodoro

PREP TIME: 10 MINUTES
COOKING TIME: 25 MINUTES
SERVES 4–6

500 g (1 lb 2 oz) penne rigate
3 tablespoons olive oil
1 onion, finely chopped
3 garlic cloves, finely chopped
3 x 400 g (14 oz) cans chopped tomatoes
1 tablespoon tomato paste (purée)
bouquet garni
3 tablespoons torn basil
freshly grated Parmesan cheese, to serve
 (optional)

NUTRITION PER SERVE (6): Fat 10.5 g; Carbohydrate 65 g;
Protein 11 g; Dietary Fibre 6 g; Cholesterol 0 mg;
1675 kJ (399 Cal)

1 Cook the pasta in a large saucepan of rapidly boiling salted water until *al dente*. Drain.

2 While the pasta is cooking, heat the oil in a deep frying pan and cook the onion over medium heat for 4–5 minutes, or until softened. Add the garlic and cook for 30 seconds before adding the tomato, tomato paste, bouquet garni and some salt and freshly ground black pepper. Reduce the heat to low and simmer for 15–20 minutes, or until the sauce thickens, stirring occasionally. Add the basil and, if the sauce is too tart, a pinch of sugar. Remove the bouquet garni. Toss the sauce through the hot pasta and serve with grated Parmesan, if desired.

penne arrabiata

PREP TIME: 5 MINUTES
COOKING TIME: 25 MINUTES
SERVES 4–6

500 g (1 lb 2 oz) penne rigate
2 tablespoons olive oil
4 garlic cloves, finely chopped
1 1/2 teaspoons chilli flakes
2 x 400 g (14 oz) cans chopped tomatoes
2 tablespoons chopped flat-leaf (Italian)
 parsley
freshly grated Parmesan cheese, to serve
 (optional)

NUTRITION PER SERVE (6): Fat 6.5 g; Carbohydrate 4.5 g;
Protein 1.5 g; Dietary Fibre 2 g; Cholesterol 0 mg;
335 kJ (80 Cal)

1 Cook the pasta in a large saucepan of rapidly boiling salted water until *al dente*. Drain.

2 While the pasta is cooking, heat the oil in a saucepan over low heat. Add the garlic and chilli flakes and cook for 3–4 minutes, or until the garlic is lightly golden. Add the tomato, season with salt and simmer for 15–20 minutes, or until reduced and thick. Stir in the parsley and season to taste.

3 Add the hot pasta to the sauce and toss through until well combined. Serve immediately, sprinkled with grated Parmesan, if desired.

pictured: pasta pomodoro

spaghetti with olive, caper and anchovy sauce

PREP TIME: 15 MINUTES
COOKING TIME: 20 MINUTES
SERVES 6

375 g (13 oz) spaghetti
4 tablespoons olive oil
2 onions, finely chopped
3 garlic cloves, finely chopped
1/2 teaspoon chilli flakes
6 large ripe tomatoes, diced
4 tablespoons capers in brine, rinsed
    and drained
7–8 anchovies in oil, drained, minced
150 g (51/2 oz) Kalamata olives
3 tablespoons chopped parsley

NUTRITION PER SERVE: Fat 15 g; Carbohydrate 49 g;
Protein 10 g; Dietary Fibre 6.5 g; Cholesterol 2 mg;
1563 kJ (373 Cal)

1 Bring a large saucepan of salted water to a boil, add the spaghetti and cook until *al dente*. Drain.

2 Meanwhile, heat the oil in a saucepan, add the onion and cook over medium heat for 5 minutes. Add the garlic and chilli flakes, and cook for 30 seconds, then add the tomato, capers and anchovies. Simmer over low heat for 5–10 minutes, or until thick and pulpy, then stir in the olives and chopped parsley.

3 Stir the pasta through the sauce. Season with salt and freshly ground black pepper and serve immediately with crusty bread.

spaghetti bolognese

PREP TIME: 30 MINUTES
COOKING TIME: 1 HOUR 20 MINUTES
SERVES 6

cooking oil spray
2 onions, finely chopped
2 cloves garlic, finely chopped
2 carrots, finely chopped
2 celery sticks, finely chopped
400 g (14 oz) lean minced (ground) beef
1 kg (21/4 lb) tomatoes, chopped
125 ml (1/2 cup) red wine
350 g (3/4 lb) spaghetti
3 tablespoons finely chopped parsley
    plus extra to garnish

NUTRITION PER SERVE: Fat 8 g; Carbohydrate 50 g;
Protein 9 g; Dietary Fibre 7 g; Cholesterol 0 mg;
1695 kJ (405 Cal)

1 Spray a large saucepan with oil. Heat over medium heat, add the onion, garlic, carrot and celery and stir for 5 minutes, or until the vegetables have softened. If you find the vegetables are sticking, add 1 tablespoon water.

2 Increase the heat to high, add the beef and stir for 5 minutes, or until browned. Add the tomato, wine and 250 ml (1 cup) water. Bring to the boil, reduce the heat and simmer, uncovered, for 1 hour, until thickened.

3 Cook the spaghetti in a large pan of rapidly boiling salted water for 10–12 minutes, or until *al dente*. Drain, stir the parsley through the sauce and season well. Divide the spaghetti among pasta bowls and top with the bolognese sauce. Garnish with parsley.

pictured: spaghetti with olive, caper
and anchovy sauce

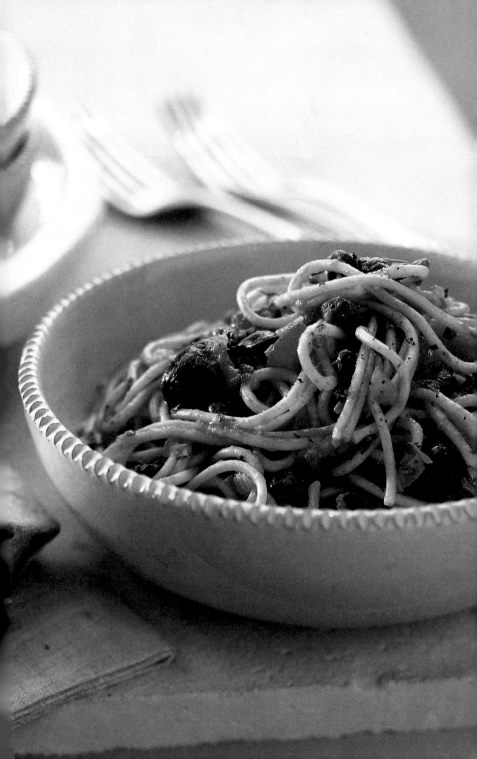

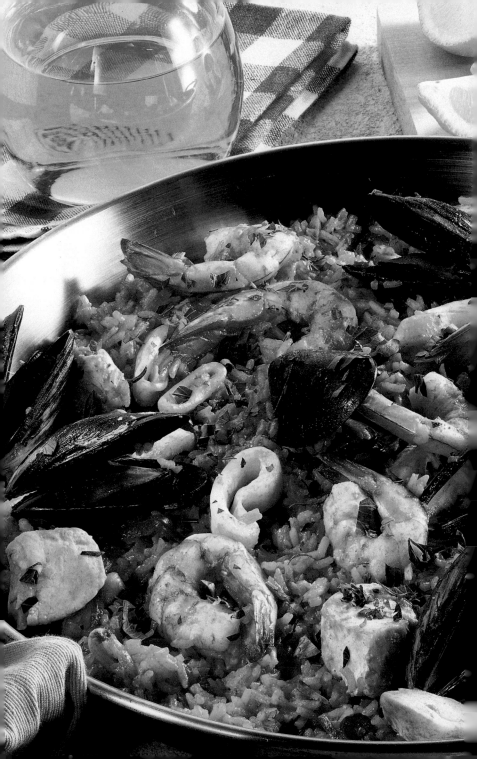

easy seafood paella

PREP TIME: 25 MINUTES
COOKING TIME: 45 MINUTES
SERVES 6

250 g (9 oz) black mussels, scrubbed,
   hairy beards removed
500 g (1 lb 2 oz) raw medium prawns
   (shrimp), peeled and deveined,
   tails intact
300 g ($10^1/_2$ oz) skinless firm white fish
   fillets such as perch or ling, cut into
   2.5 cm (1 inch) cubes
200 g (7 oz) squid rings
3 tablespoons olive oil
1 large onion, diced
3 garlic cloves, finely chopped
1 small red capsicum (pepper),
   thinly sliced
1 small red chilli, deseeded and
   chopped, optional
2 teaspoons paprika
1 teaspoon ground turmeric
2 tomatoes, peeled and diced
1 tablespoon tomato paste (purée)
400 g (2 cups) long-grain rice
125 ml ($^1/_2$ cup) white wine
1.25 litres (5 cups) fish stock
3 tablespoons chopped parsley, to serve
lemon wedges, to serve

NUTRITION PER SERVE: Fat 14.5 g; Carbohydrate 58.5 g;
Protein 44.5 g; Dietary Fibre 3.5 g; Cholesterol 217 mg;
2360 kJ (560 Cal)

note: You can use just fish, or other seafood such as scampi, octopus, crabs. If using just fish, choose one with few bones and chunky flesh, such as ling, blue eye or warehou.

1 Discard any broken mussels or those that don't close when tapped. Keep the seafood in the fridge, covered, until ready to use.

2 Heat the oil in a paella pan or a large deep frying pan (about 32 cm/13 inch diameter) with a lid. Add the onion, garlic, capsicum and chilli to the pan and cook over medium heat for 2 minutes, or until the onion and capsicum are soft. Add the paprika, turmeric and 1 teaspoon salt and stir-fry for 1–2 minutes, or until aromatic. Add the tomato and cook for 5 minutes, or until soft. Add the tomato paste. Stir in the rice until well coated.

3 Pour in the white wine and simmer until almost absorbed. Add the stock, bring to a boil, then reduce the heat and simmer for 20 minutes, or until almost all the liquid is absorbed into the rice. Fluff up the rice occasionally with a fork to separate the grains.

4 Add the mussels to the pan, poking the shells into the rice, cover and cook for 2–3 minutes over low heat. Add the prawns and cook for 2–3 minutes. Add the fish, cover and cook for 3 minutes. Add the squid rings and cook for 1–2 minutes. By this time, the mussels should have opened—discard any unopened ones. The prawns should be pink and the fish should flake easily when tested with a fork. The squid should be white and tender. Cook for another 2–3 minutes if the seafood is not cooked, but avoid overcooking as the seafood will toughen and dry out.

5 Serve with parsley and lemon wedges. Delicious with a tossed salad.

moroccan vegetable stew with minty couscous

PREP TIME: 25 MINUTES + 5 MINUTES
   STANDING
COOKING TIME: 50 MINUTES
SERVES 4

2 tablespoons olive oil
1 onion, finely chopped
3 garlic cloves, finely chopped
1 teaspoon ground ginger
1 teaspoon ground turmeric
2 teaspoons ground cumin
2 teaspoons ground cinnamon
1/2 teaspoon dried chilli flakes
400 g (14 oz) can chopped tomatoes
400 g (14 oz) can chickpeas, rinsed
   and drained
80 g (1/2 cup) sultanas
400 g (14 oz) butternut pumpkin (squash),
   cut into 3 cm (1 1/4 inch) cubes
2 large zucchini (courgettes), cut into
   2 cm (3/4 inch) pieces
2 carrots, cut into 2 cm (3/4 inch) pieces
185 g (1 cup) instant couscous
25 g (1 oz) butter
4 tablespoons chopped mint

NUTRITION PER SERVE: Fat 14 g; Carbohydrate 75 g;
Protein 15 g; Dietary Fibre 12 g; Cholesterol 0 mg;
2024 kJ (484 Cal)

1 Heat the olive oil in a large saucepan over medium heat. Add the onion and cook for 3–5 minutes, or until translucent but not brown. Add the garlic, ginger, turmeric, cumin, cinnamon and chilli flakes and cook for 1 minute. Add the tomato, chickpeas, sultanas and 250 ml (1 cup) water. Bring to the boil, then reduce the heat and simmer, covered, for 20 minutes. Add the pumpkin, zucchini and carrot and cook for another 20 minutes, or until the vegetables are tender. Season with salt and ground black pepper.

2 Place the couscous in a large, heatproof bowl. Cover with 250 ml (1 cup) boiling water and leave to stand for 5 minutes, or until all the water is absorbed. Fluff with a fork and stir in the butter and mint. Season with salt and freshly ground black pepper, and serve with the stew.

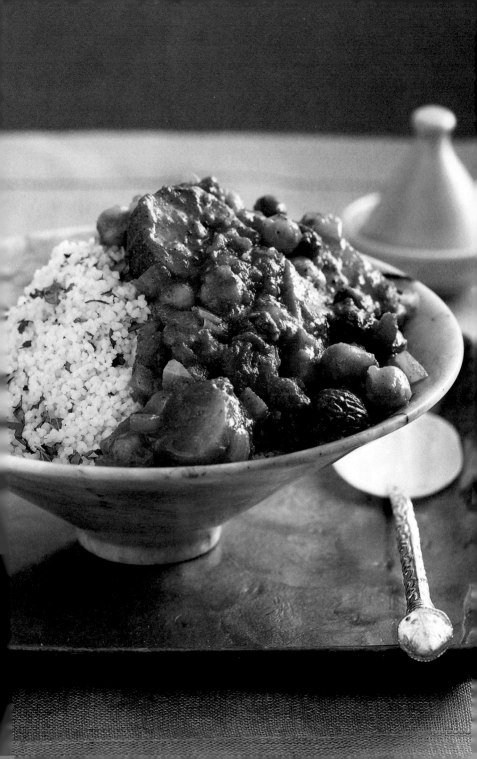

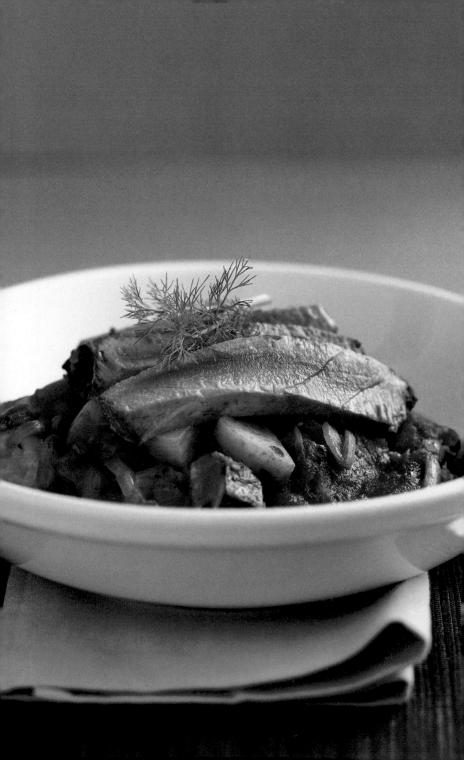

tuna with potato ratatouille

PREP TIME: 15 MINUTES
COOKING TIME: 1 HOUR
SERVES 4

3 tablespoons olive oil
1 teaspoon grated lemon zest
4 garlic cloves, crushed
4 x 175 g (6 oz) pieces of tuna
1 red onion, thinly sliced
350 g ($^3/_4$ lb) fennel, thinly sliced
125 ml ($^1/_2$ cup) dry white wine
830 g (1 lb 13 oz) canned chopped
    tomatoes
600 g (1 lb 5 oz) new potatoes, quartered
350 g ($^3/_4$ lb) zucchini (courgettes), cut into
    1.5 cm ($^5/_8$ inch) rounds
2 tablespoons lemon juice
2 tablespoons chopped parsley
sprigs of fennel, to garnish

NUTRITION PER SERVE: Fat 5 g; Carbohydrate 33 g; Protein 38 g; Dietary Fibre 10 g; Cholesterol 50 mg; 1400 kJ (333 Cal)

1 Combine 1 tablespoon of the oil with the lemon zest and half the garlic. Place the tuna in a flat dish and cover with the marinade. Refrigerate.

2 Heat 1 tablespoon oil in a saucepan, add the onion and cook for 5 minutes, or until soft. Add the fennel and remaining garlic and cook, stirring, over low heat for 15–20 minutes, or until softened. Increase the heat to medium, stir in the white wine and cook for 2 minutes.

3 Add the tomato and potato, bring to a boil, then reduce the heat and simmer for 20 minutes, or until the potato is tender. Add the zucchini and cook for 5 minutes, or until tender. Season and stir in the parsley. Remove from the heat and keep warm.

4 Heat the remaining oil in a large non-stick frying pan. Cook the tuna for 1–2 minutes each side. Add the lemon juice and cook for 20–30 seconds. Remove from the pan, cool slightly and cut into 2 cm ($^3/_4$ inch) slices. Serve the ratatouille with the tuna slices over the top. Garnish with the fennel sprigs.

blue eye with spicy tomato sauce

PREP TIME: 5 MINUTES
COOKING TIME: 25 MINUTES
SERVES 4

4 blue eye cutlets, 2.5 cm (1 inch) thick
    (about 250 g/9 oz each)
250 g (1¼ cups) long-grain rice
2 tablespoons oil
1 teaspoon coriander seeds, lightly
    crushed
1 teaspoon black mustard seeds
1½ tablespoons sambal oelek
400 g (14 oz) can chopped tomatoes
1 teaspoon garam masala
300 g (10½ oz) baby English spinach
    leaves

NUTRITION PER SERVE: Fat 12 g; Carbohydrate 56 g;
Protein 50.5 g; Dietary Fibre 4.5 g; Cholesterol 130 mg;
2245 kJ (535 Cal)

1 Preheat the oven to 180°C (350°F/Gas 4). Pat the cutlets dry with paper towels.

2 Bring a large saucepan of water to a boil. Add the rice and cook for 12 minutes, stirring occasionally with a fork. Drain well.

3 Meanwhile, heat 1 tablespoon of the oil in a saucepan over medium heat. When hot, add the coriander and mustard seeds—the mustard seeds should start to pop after about 30 seconds. Add the sambal oelek and cook for 30 seconds, then stir in the tomato and garam masala. Bring to the boil, then reduce the heat to low and simmer, covered, for 6–8 minutes, or until the sauce thickens.

4 Heat the remaining oil in a large non-stick frying pan over medium heat. Add the cutlets and cook for 1 minute each side, or until evenly browned but not cooked through. Transfer to a 28 x 18 cm (10 x 7 inch) ceramic baking dish. Spoon the tomato sauce over the cutlets and bake for 10 minutes, or until the fish is cooked through.

5 Meanwhile, wash the spinach and put in a saucepan with just the water clinging to the leaves. Cook, covered, for 1 minute, or until the spinach has wilted. Serve the fish cutlets topped with sauce, with the spinach and some steamed rice.

note: Sambal oelek is available form Asian shops and some supermarkets.

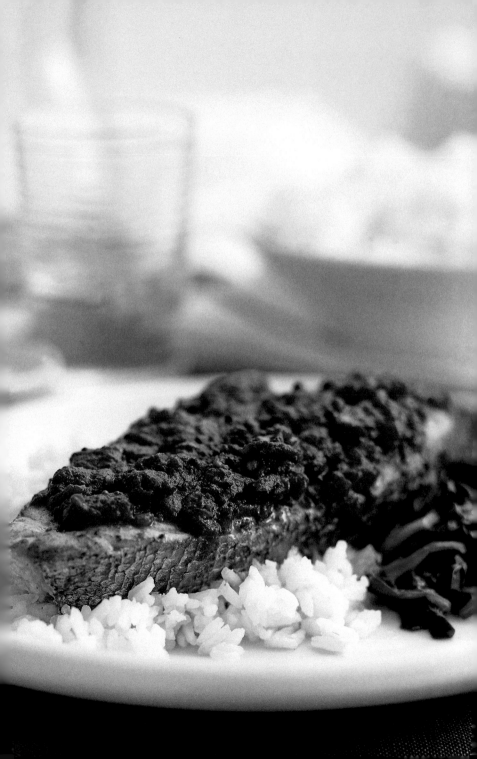

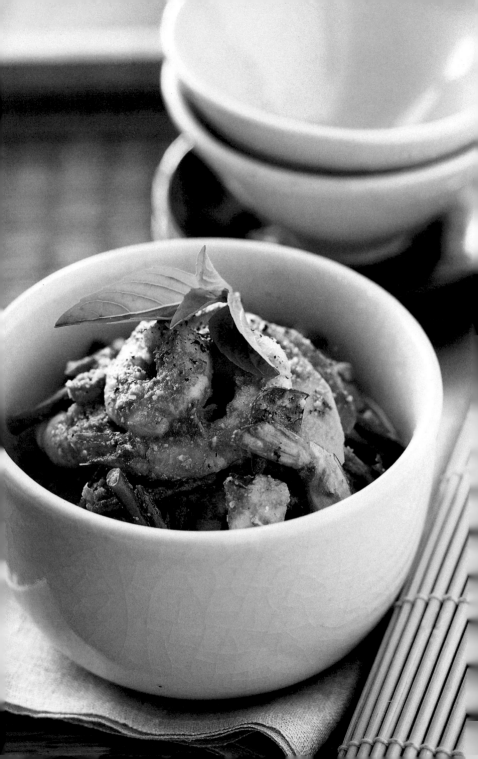

jungle curry prawns

PREP TIME: 30 MINUTES + 15 MINUTES
  SOAKING
COOKING TIME: 10 MINUTES
SERVES 6

Curry paste

10–12 large dried red chillies
1 teaspoon white pepper
4 red Asian shallots
4 garlic cloves, sliced
1 stem lemon grass, white part only, sliced
1 tablespoon finely chopped galangal
2 small coriander (cilantro) roots, chopped
1 tablespoon finely chopped fresh ginger
1 tablespoon shrimp paste, dry roasted

1 tablespoon peanut oil
1 garlic clove, crushed
1 tablespoon fish sauce
30 g ($1/4$ cup) ground macadamia nuts
315 ml ($1 1/4$ cups) fish stock
1 tablespoon whisky
3 fresh kaffir lime leaves, torn
600 g (1 lb 5 oz) raw prawns (shrimp),
  peeled, deveined and tails intact
1 small carrot, quartered lengthways
  and sliced thinly on the diagonal
150 g ($5 1/2$ oz) snake beans, cut into
  2 cm ($3/4$ inch) lengths
50 g ($1 3/4$ oz) bamboo shoots
Thai basil leaves, to garnish

NUTRITION PER SERVE: Fat 7 g; Carbohydrate 2.5 g;
Protein 23 g; Dietary Fibre 2.5 g; Cholesterol 150 mg;
725 kJ (173 Cal)

1 To make the curry paste, soak the chillies in boiling water for 15 minutes, then drain and chop. Transfer to a food processor and add the white pepper, shallots, garlic, lemon grass, galangal, coriander roots, ginger, shrimp paste and 1 teaspoon salt. Blend until smooth, adding a little water if necessary.

2 Heat a wok over medium heat, add the oil and swirl to coat. Add the garlic and 3 tablespoons of the curry paste and cook, stirring, for 5 minutes. Add the fish sauce, ground macadamia nuts, fish stock, whisky, kaffir lime leaves, prawns, carrot, beans and bamboo shoots. Bring to the boil, then reduce the heat and simmer for 5 minutes, or until the prawns and vegetables are cooked.

3 Garnish with Thai basil and freshly ground black pepper.

cajun chicken with fresh tomato and corn salsa

PREP TIME: 15 MINUTES
COOKING TIME: 15 MINUTES
SERVES 4

2 corn cobs
2 vine-ripened tomatoes, diced
1 Lebanese (short) cucumber, diced
2 tablespoons roughly chopped coriander
  (cilantro)
4 chicken breast fillets
  (about 200 g/7 oz each)
35 g (^{1}/4 cup) Cajun seasoning (see Note)
2 tablespoons lime juice
lime wedges, to serve

NUTRITION PER SERVE: Fat 7 g; Carbohydrate 16.5 g; Protein 26 g; Dietary Fibre 5 g; Cholesterol 66 mg; 980 kJ (235 Cal)

1 Cook the corn cobs in a saucepan of boiling water for 5 minutes, or until tender. Scrape off the kernels using a sharp knife and put them in a bowl with the tomato, cucumber and chopped coriander. Season, to taste, and mix well.

2 Heat a chargrill pan (griddle) or barbecue plate to medium heat and brush lightly with oil.

3 Pound each chicken breast between two sheets of plastic wrap with a mallet or rolling pin until 2 cm (^{3}/4 inch) thick. Lightly coat the chicken with the Cajun seasoning and shake off any excess. Cook for 5 minutes on each side, or until just cooked through.

4 Just before serving, stir the lime juice into the salsa. Place a chicken breast on each plate and spoon the salsa on the side. Serve with the lime wedges. Delicious with a green salad and crusty bread.

note: Cajun seasoning is available from the spice section of supermarkets.

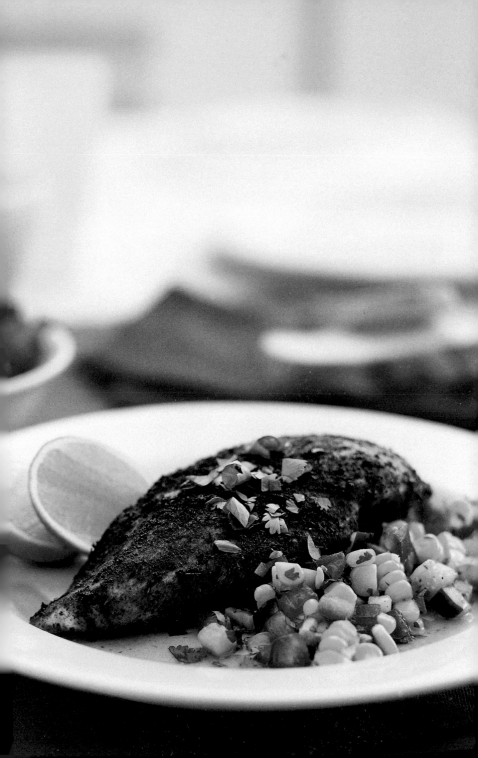

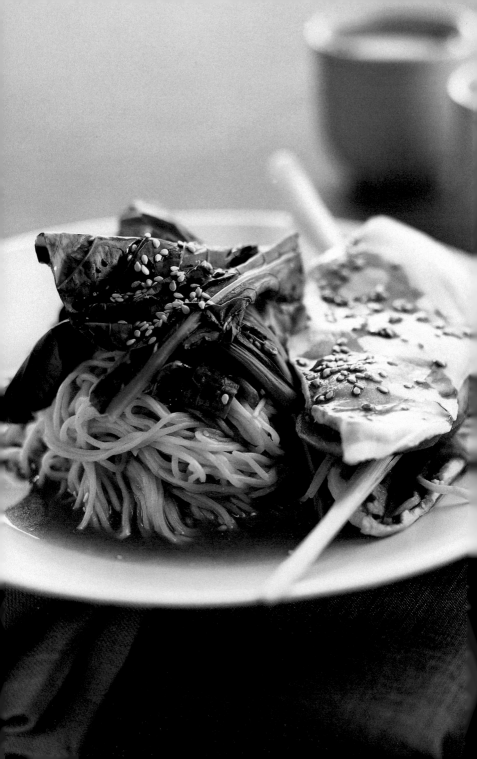

steamed lemon grass and ginger chicken with Asian greens

PREP TIME: 25 MINUTES
COOKING TIME: 40 MINUTES
SERVES 4

200 g (7 oz) fresh egg noodles
4 chicken breast fillets
2 stems lemon grass
5 cm (2 inch) piece fresh ginger, cut into
     julienne strips
1 lime, thinly sliced
500 ml (2 cups) chicken stock
1 bunch (350 g) choy sum, cut into
     10 cm (4 inch) lengths
800 g (1 3/4 lb) Chinese broccoli, cut into
     10 cm (4 inch) lengths
3 tablespoons kecap manis
60 ml (1/4 cup) soy sauce
1 teaspoon sesame oil
toasted sesame seeds, to garnish

NUTRITION PER SERVE: Fat 7.5 g; Carbohydrate 37 g; Protein 65 g; Dietary Fibre 9 g; Cholesterol 119 mg; 2045 kJ (488 Cal)

1 Cook the fresh egg noodles in a saucepan of boiling water for 5 minutes, then drain and keep warm.

2 Cut each chicken breast fillet horizontally through the middle to make eight thin flat chicken fillets.

3 Cut the lemon grass into lengths that are about 5 cm (2 inches) longer than the chicken fillets, then cut in half lengthways. Place one piece of lemon grass onto one half of each chicken breast fillet, top with some ginger and lime slices, then top with the other half of the fillet.

4 Pour the stock into a wok and bring to a simmer. Place two of the chicken fillets in a paper-lined bamboo steamer. Place the steamer over the wok and steam over the simmering stock for 12–15 minutes, or until the chicken is tender. Remove the chicken from the steamer, cover and keep warm. Repeat with the other fillets.

5 Steam the greens in the same way for 3 minutes, or until tender. Bring the stock in the wok to a boil.

6 Place the kecap manis, soy sauce and sesame oil in a bowl and whisk together well.

7 Divide the noodles among four serving plates and ladle the boiling stock over them. Top with a neat pile of Asian greens, then add the chicken and generously drizzle each serve with the sauce. Garnish with toasted sesame seeds and serve immediately.

chicken in creamy tomato sauce

PREP TIME: 35 MINUTES
COOKING TIME: 1 HOUR 40 MINUTES
SERVES 8–10

1 tablespoon oil
2 x 1.5 kg (3 lb 5 oz) chickens, jointed
1 onion, sliced
1/2 teaspoon ground cloves
1 teaspoon ground turmeric
2 teaspoons garam masala
3 teaspoons chilli powder
3 garlic cloves
1 tablespoon finely chopped fresh ginger
1 tablespoon poppy seeds
2 teaspoons fennel seeds
3 cardamom pods, seeds removed
    (see Note)
250 ml (1 cup) coconut milk
1 star anise
1 cinnamon stick
4 large tomatoes, roughly chopped
2 tablespoons lime juice

NUTRITION PER SERVE (10): Fat 11 g; Carbohydrate 6.5 g;
Protein 35 g; Dietary Fibre 1.5 g; Cholesterol 75 mg;
1027 kJ (245 Cal)

1 Heat the oil in a large frying pan, add the chicken in batches and cook for 5–10 minutes, or until browned, then transfer to a large saucepan.

2 Add the onion to the frying pan and cook, stirring, for 10–12 minutes, or until golden. Stir in the cloves, turmeric, garam masala and chilli powder and cook, stirring, for a minute, then add to the chicken.

3 Process the garlic, ginger, poppy seeds, fennel seeds, cardamom seeds and 2 tablespoons of the coconut milk in a food processor or blender until smooth. Add the spice mixture, remaining coconut milk, star anise, cinnamon stick, tomato and 3 tablespoons water to the chicken.

4 Simmer, covered, for 45 minutes, or until the chicken is tender. Remove the chicken, cover and keep warm. Bring the cooking liquid to a boil and boil for 20–25 minutes, or until reduced by half. Place the chicken on a serving plate, mix the lime juice with the cooking liquid and pour over the chicken. Serve with plain yoghurt.

note: To remove the cardamom seeds from the cardamom pods, crush the pods with the flat side of a heavy knife, then peel away the pod with your fingers, scraping out the seeds.

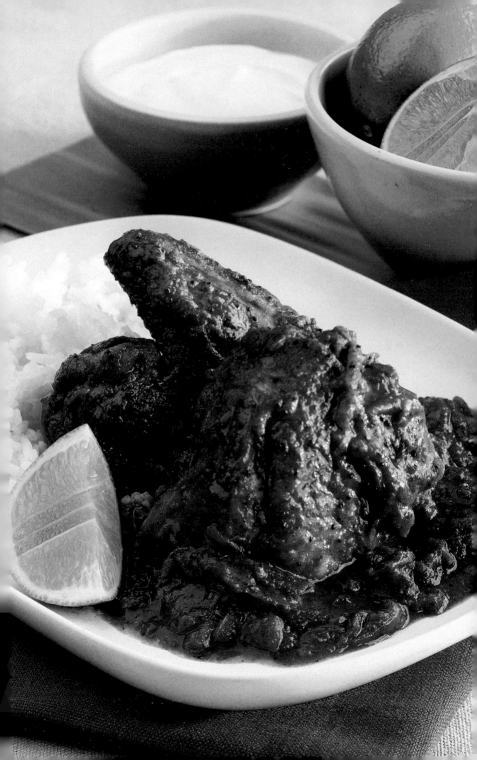

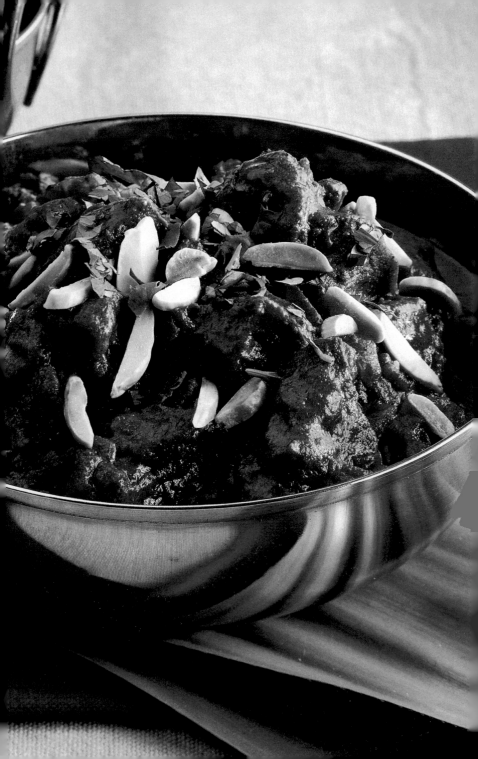

rogan josh

PREP TIME: 25 MINUTES
COOKING TIME: 1 HOUR 40 MINUTES
SERVES 4–6

1 kg (2^1/$_4$ lb) boned leg of lamb
1 tablespoon ghee or oil
2 onions, chopped
125 g (^{1}/$_2$ cup) plain yoghurt
1 teaspoon chilli powder
1 tablespoon ground coriander
2 teaspoons ground cumin
1 teaspoon ground cardamom
^{1}/$_2$ teaspoon ground cloves
1 teaspoon ground turmeric
3 garlic cloves, crushed
1 tablespoon grated fresh ginger
400 g (14 oz) can chopped tomatoes
30 g (^{1}/$_4$ cup) slivered almonds
1 teaspoon garam masala
chopped coriander (cilantro), to garnish

NUTRITION PER SERVE (6): Fat 13 g; Carbohydrate 5.5 g;
Protein 40 g; Dietary Fibre 2 g; Cholesterol 122 mg;
1236 kJ (295 Cal)

1 Trim the lamb of any excess fat or sinew and cut into 2.5 cm (1 inch) cubes.

2 Heat the ghee in a large saucepan, add the onion and cook, stirring, for 5 minutes, or until soft. Stir in the yoghurt, chilli powder, coriander, cumin, cardamom, cloves, turmeric, garlic and ginger. Add the chopped tomato and 1 teaspoon salt, then simmer for 5 minutes.

3 Add the lamb and stir until coated. Cover and cook over low heat, stirring occasionally, for 1–1^1/$_2$ hours, or until the lamb is tender. Uncover and simmer until the liquid thickens.

4 Meanwhile, toast the almonds in a dry frying pan over medium heat for 3–4 minutes, shaking the pan gently, until the nuts are golden brown. Remove from the pan at once to prevent them burning.

5 Add the garam masala to the curry and mix through well. Sprinkle the slivered almonds and chopped coriander over the top and serve.

hearty pork stew

PREP TIME: 15 MINUTES + OVERNIGHT
  MARINATING
COOKING TIME: 1 HOUR 20 MINUTES
SERVES 4–6

1¹/₂ tablespoons coriander seeds
800 g (1³/₄ lb) pork fillet, cut into
  2 cm (³/₄ inch) dice
1 tablespoon plain (all-purpose) flour
3 tablespoons olive oil
1 large onion, thinly sliced
375 ml (1¹/₂ cups) red wine
250 ml (1 cup) chicken stock
1 teaspoon sugar
coriander (cilantro) sprigs, to garnish

NUTRITION PER SERVE (6): Fat 12 g; Carbohydrate 2.5 g;
Protein 30 g; Dietary Fibre 0 g; Cholesterol 65 mg;
1180 kJ (282 Cal)

1 Crush the coriander seeds in a mortar and pestle. Combine the pork, crushed seeds and ¹/₂ teaspoon cracked pepper in a bowl. Cover and marinate overnight in the fridge.

2 Toss the flour with the pork. Heat 2 tablespoons of the oil in a frying pan and cook the pork in batches over high heat for 1–2 minutes, or until brown. Remove from the pan.

3 Heat the remaining oil in the frying pan, add the onion and cook over medium heat for 2–3 minutes, or until just golden. Return the meat to the pan, add the red wine, chicken stock and sugar, then season to taste. Bring to a boil, then reduce the heat and simmer, covered, for 1 hour.

4 Remove the meat from the pan with a slotted spoon. Return the pan to the heat and boil the liquid over a high heat for 3–5 minutes, or until reduced and slightly thickened. Pour the sauce over the meat and garnish with the coriander sprigs.

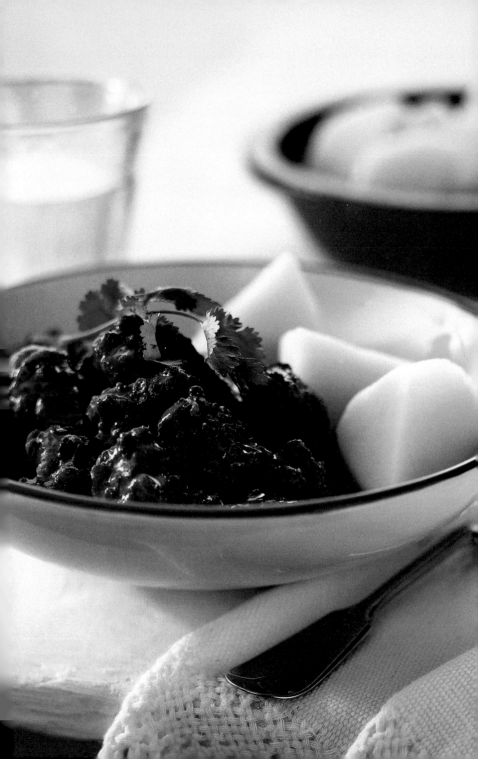

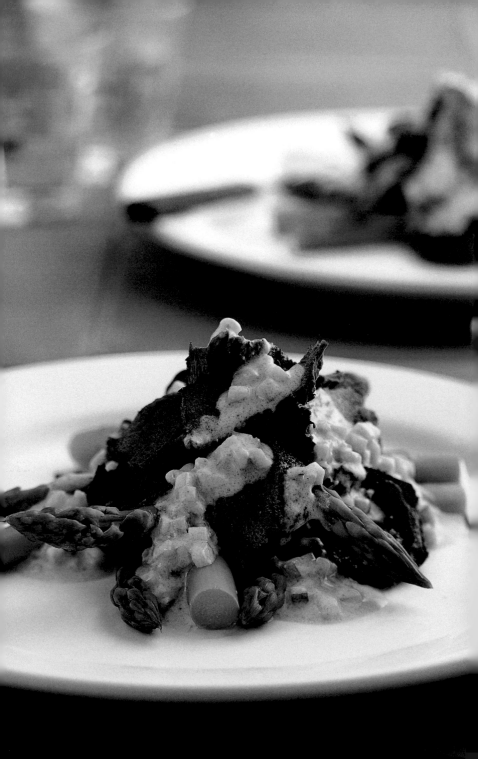

lamb with roasted tomatoes

PREP TIME: 20 MINUTES
COOKING TIME: 1 HOUR 10 MINUTES
SERVES 4–6

1 tablespoon red wine vinegar
1/2 Lebanese (short) cucumber, finely diced
100 g (3 1/2 oz) Greek-style yoghurt
2 teaspoons chopped mint
1/2 teaspoon ground cumin
4 tablespoons olive oil
6 vine-ripened tomatoes
4 garlic cloves, finely chopped
1 tablespoon chopped oregano
1 tablespoon chopped parsley
600 g (1 lb 5 oz) asparagus, trimmed
2 lamb backstraps or loin fillets (500 g/
    1 lb 2 oz)

NUTRITION PER SERVE (6): Fat 15 g; Carbohydrate 7 g;
Protein 26 g; Dietary Fibre 4 g; Cholesterol 59.5 mg;
1100 kJ (265 Cal)

1 Put the vinegar, cucumber, yoghurt, mint, cumin and 1 tablespoon of the olive oil in a small jug and mix well.

2 Preheat the oven to 180°C (350°F/ Gas 4). Cut the tomatoes in half and scoop out the seeds. Combine the garlic, oregano and parsley, and sprinkle into the tomato shells.

3 Place the tomatoes on a rack in a baking tin. Drizzle them with 1 tablespoon of the olive oil and roast for 1 hour. Remove from the oven, cut each piece in half again and keep warm. Place the asparagus in the roasting tin, drizzle with another tablespoon of the olive oil, season and roast for 10 minutes.

4 Meanwhile, heat the remaining oil in a frying pan. Season the lamb well and cook over medium–high heat for 5 minutes on each side, then set aside to rest.

5 Remove the asparagus from the oven and arrange on a serving plate. Top with the tomato. Slice the lamb on the diagonal and arrange on top of the tomato. Drizzle with the dressing and serve immediately.

caramel pork and pumpkin stir-fry

PREPARATION TIME: 15 MINUTES
COOKING TIME: 20 MINUTES
SERVES 4

250 g (1 1/4 cups) jasmine rice
300 g (10 1/2 oz) butternut pumpkin
   (squash)
500 g (1 lb 2 oz) pork fillet
2 garlic cloves, crushed
2–3 tablespoons peanut oil
60 g (1/3 cup) soft brown sugar
3 tablespoons fish sauce
3 tablespoons rice vinegar (see Note)
2 tablespoons chopped coriander
   (cilantro) leaves
1.25 kg (2 3/4 lb) mixed Asian greens
   such as bok choy (pak choi), choy sum,
   gai lan (Chinese broccoli)

NUTRITION PER SERVE: Fat 15 g; Carbohydrate 73 g;
Protein 38 g; Dietary Fibre 6 g; Cholesterol 118.5 mg;
2445 kJ (585 Cal)

1 Bring a large saucepan of water to the boil, add the rice and cook for 12 minutes, stirring occasionally. Drain well.

2 Meanwhile, cut the pumpkin into pieces roughly 2 x 4 cm (3/4 x 1 1/2 inch) and 5 mm (1/4 inch) thick. Thinly slice the pork, then combine with the garlic and 2 teaspoons of the peanut oil. Season with salt and plenty of pepper.

3 Heat a wok until very hot, add 1 tablespoon oil and swirl to coat. When just starting to smoke, stir-fry the pork in two batches for about 1 minute per batch, or until the meat changes colour. Transfer to a plate. Add the remaining oil to the wok and stir-fry the pumpkin for 4 minutes, or until tender but not falling apart. Remove and add to the pork.

4 Combine the sugar, fish sauce, rice vinegar and 125 ml (1/2 cup) water in the wok and boil for about 10 minutes, or until syrupy. Return the pork and pumpkin to the wok and stir for 1 minute, or until well coated and heated through. Stir in the coriander.

5 Cook the mixed Asian greens in a paper-lined bamboo steamer over a wok of simmering water for 3 minutes, or until wilted. Serve immediately with the stir-fry and rice.

note: Rice vinegar is available in the Asian section of most supermarkets.

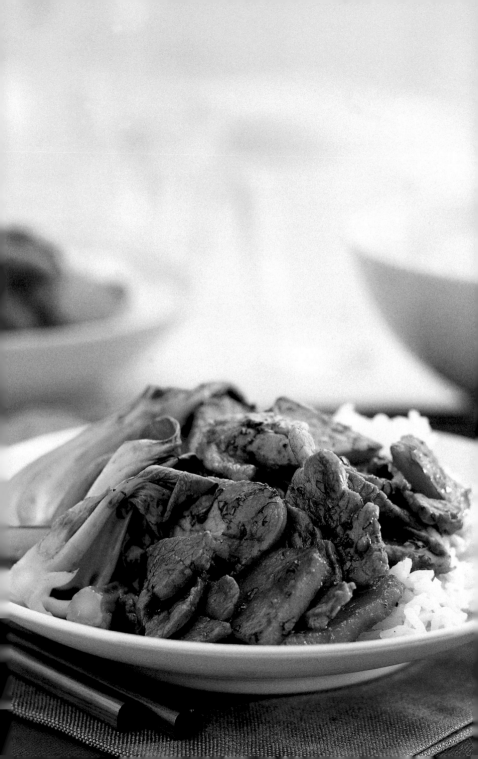

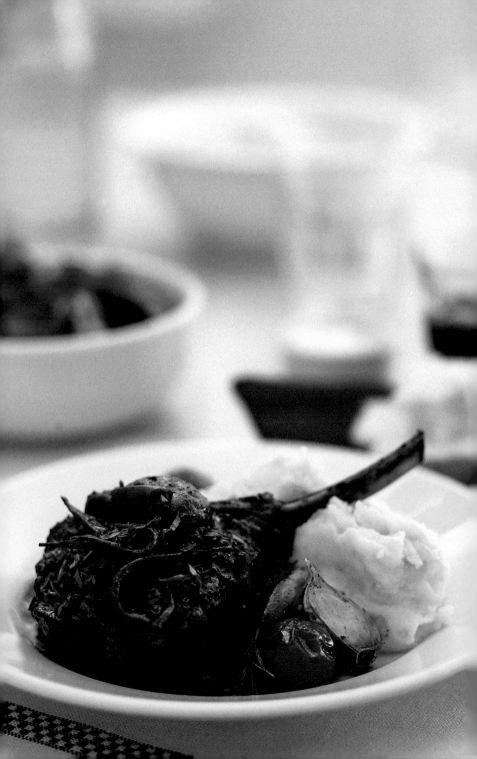

balsamic roasted veal cutlets with red onion

PREP TIME: 10 MINUTES
COOKING TIME: 45 MINUTES
SERVES 4

1^1/$_2$ tablespoons olive oil
8 veal cutlets
4 garlic cloves, unpeeled
1 red onion, cut into thin wedges
1 tablespoon chopped rosemary
250 g (9 oz) cherry tomatoes
3 tablespoons balsamic vinegar
2 teaspoons soft brown sugar
2 tablespoons chopped parsley, to garnish

NUTRITION PER SERVE: Fat 11 g; Carbohydrate 5 g; Protein 41 g; Dietary Fibre 2 g; Cholesterol 146 mg; 1200 kJ (285 Cal)

1 Preheat the oven to 200°C (400°F/ Gas 6). Heat the oil in a large frying pan over medium heat. Cook the cutlets in batches for 4 minutes on both sides, or until brown.

2 Arrange the cutlets in a single layer in a large, shallow roasting tin. Add the garlic, onion, rosemary, tomatoes, vinegar and sugar. Season well with salt and black pepper.

3 Cover the tin tightly with foil and roast for 15 minutes. Remove the foil and roast for another 10–15 minutes, depending on the thickness of the veal cutlets.

4 Transfer the cutlets, garlic, onion and tomatoes to serving plates. Stir the pan juices and spoon over the top. Garnish with the chopped parsley and serve immediately. Delicious with a creamy garlic mash and a green salad.

index